# DIABETES

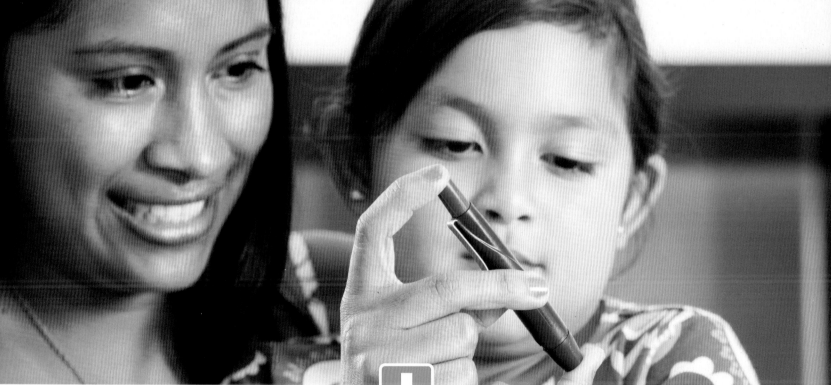

## IN CASE OF EMERGENCY

Linda Hopkins

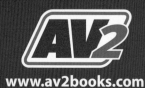

www.av2books.com

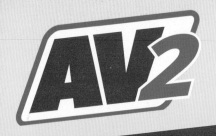

## Step 1
Go to **www.av2books.com**

## Step 2
Enter this unique code

**NPLVO7ADC**

## Step 3
Explore your interactive eBook!

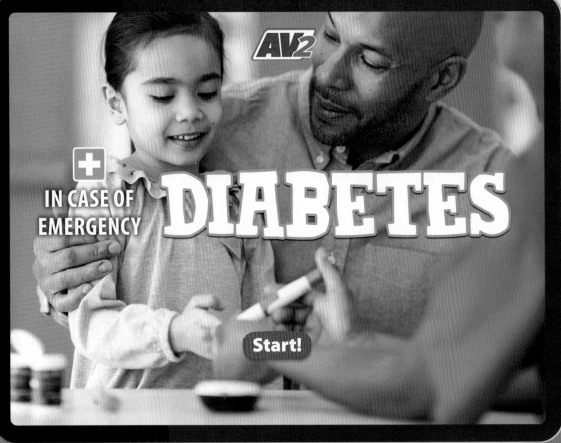

IN CASE OF EMERGENCY

**DIABETES**

**Start!**

**AV2 is optimized for use on any device**

# Your interactive eBook comes with...

**Read**

**Audio**
Listen to the entire book read aloud

**Videos**
Watch informative video clips

**Weblinks**
Gain additional information for research

**Try This!**
Complete activities and hands-on experiments

**Key Words**
Study vocabulary, and complete a matching word activity

**Quizzes**
Test your knowledge

**Slideshows**
View images and captions

# View new titles and product videos at
# www.av2books.com

## IN CASE OF EMERGENCY

# DIABETES

## Contents

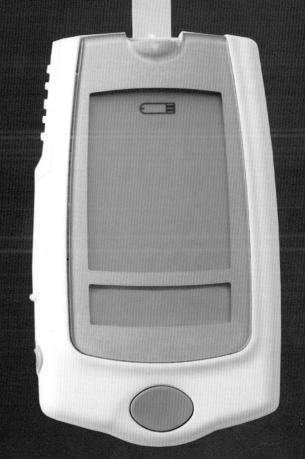

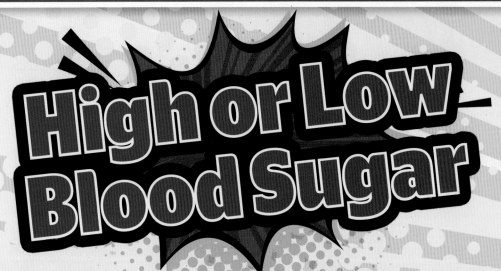

## High or Low Blood Sugar

Some people have diabetes.

With diabetes, the body struggles to get the energy it needs from food.

Diabetes can cause high or low blood sugar levels.

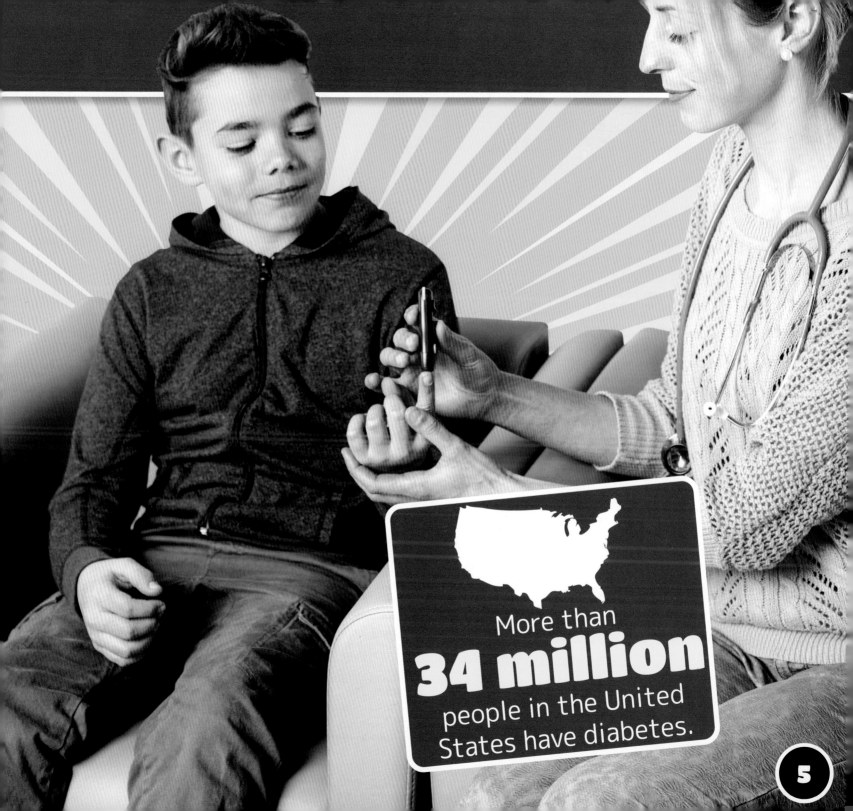

More than **34 million** people in the United States have diabetes.

# Signs and Symptoms

Low blood sugar will make a person hungry and shaky.

High blood sugar may lead to thirst, headaches, and trouble seeing.

Both high and low blood sugar can cause confusion.

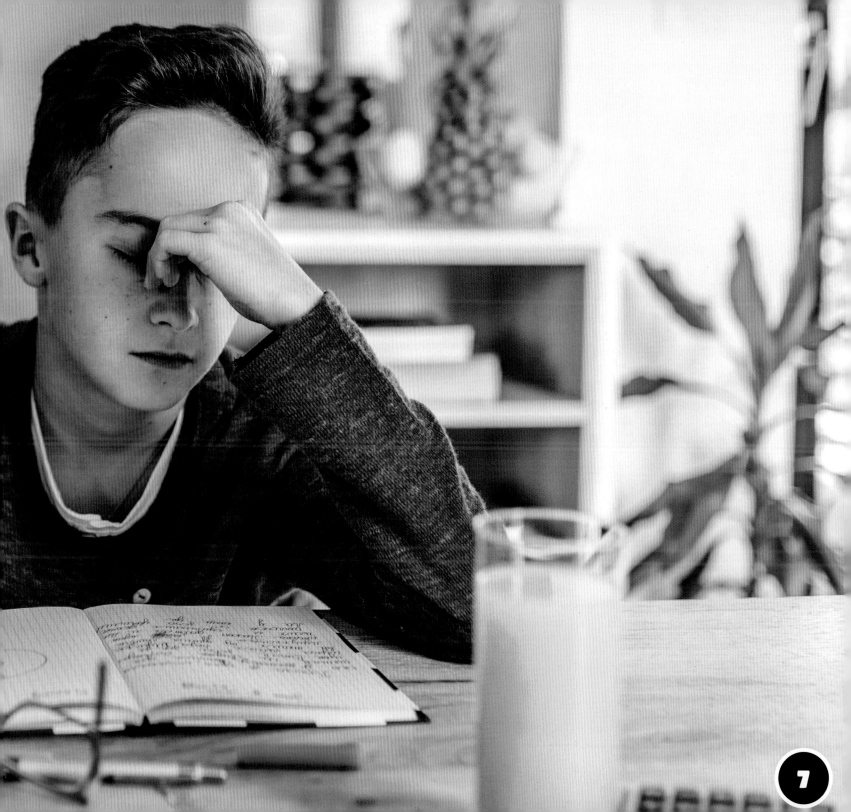

# Stay Calm

It is important to stay calm when someone is experiencing low blood sugar.

The person may feel dizzy or confused.

He or she might need your help.

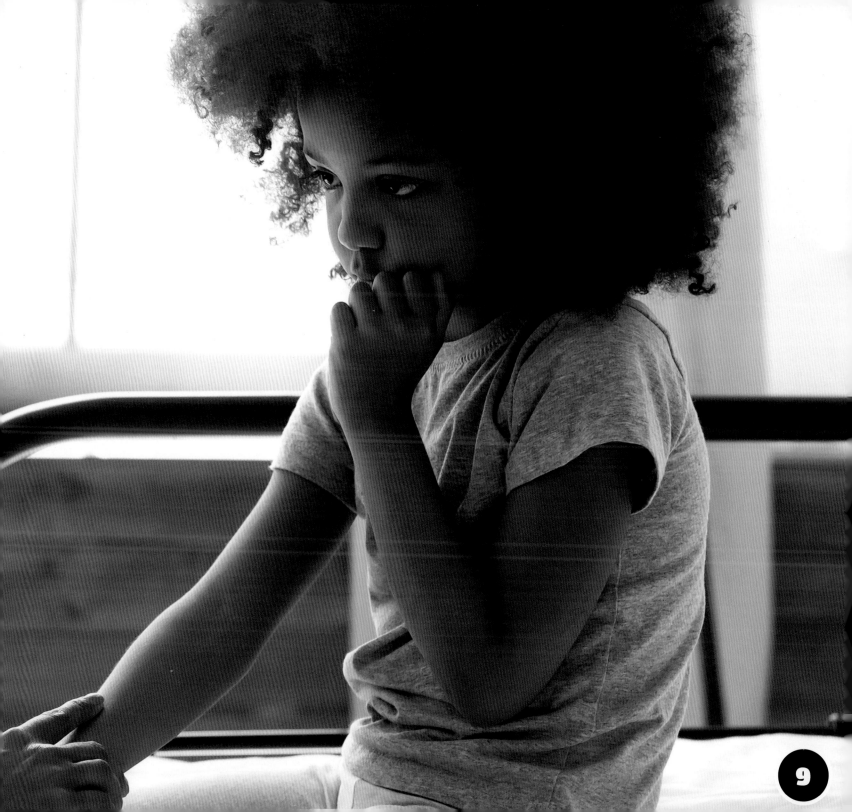

# Call 9-1-1

Call 9-1-1 if the person faints.

The 9-1-1 operator will need to know your name, where you are, and what the emergency is.

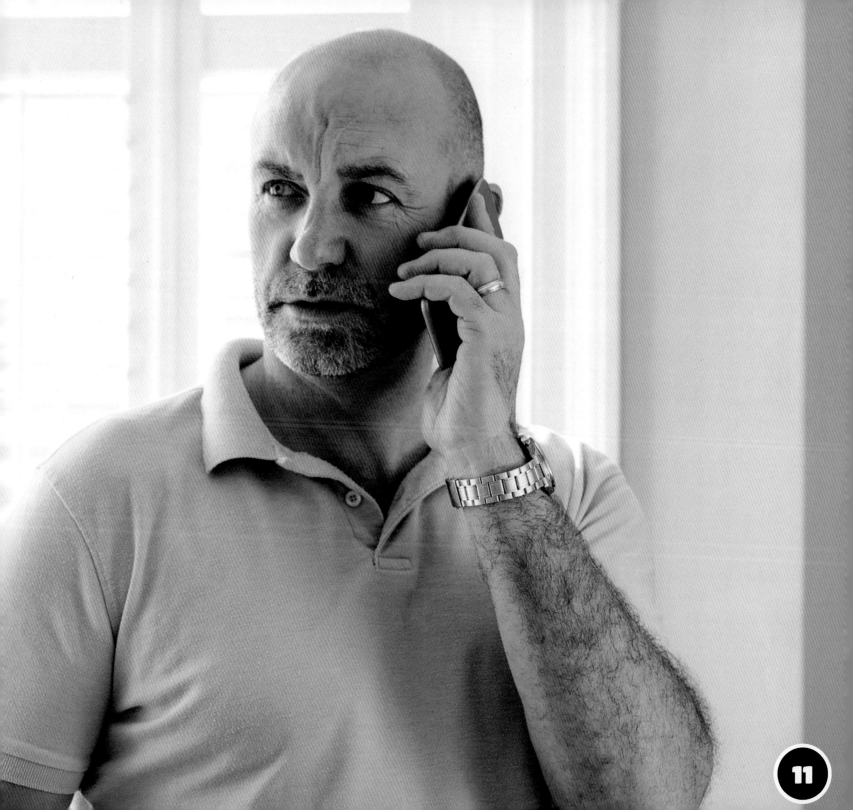

# Sit Down

Someone with low blood sugar should sit down.

Walking or moving can make blood sugar drop lower.

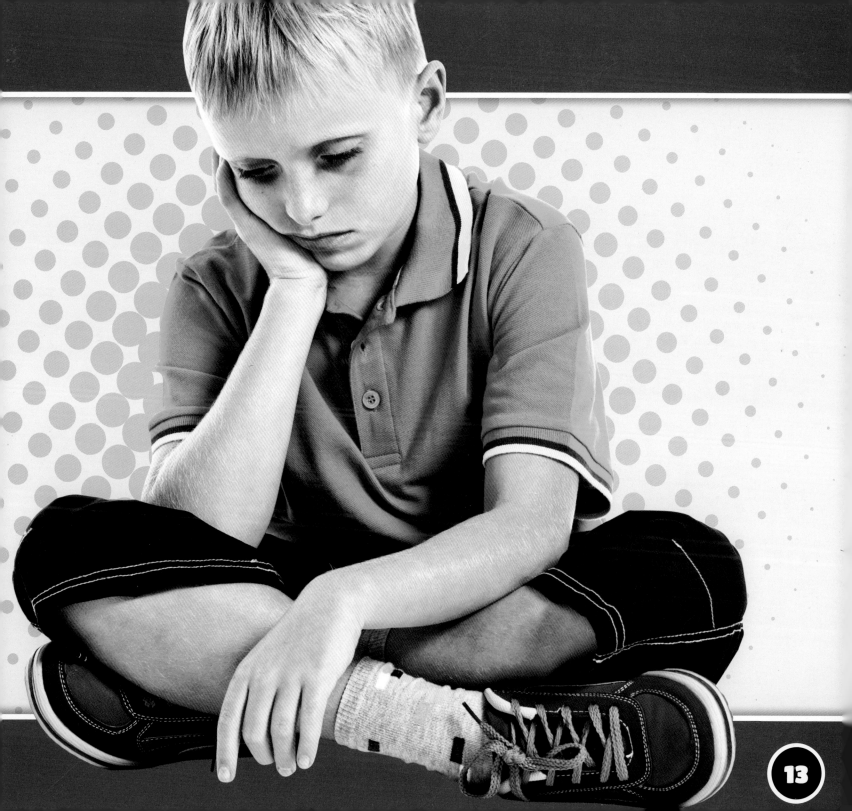

## Take Sugar

A person with low blood sugar should eat or drink a sugary snack.

Offer the person juice or candy.

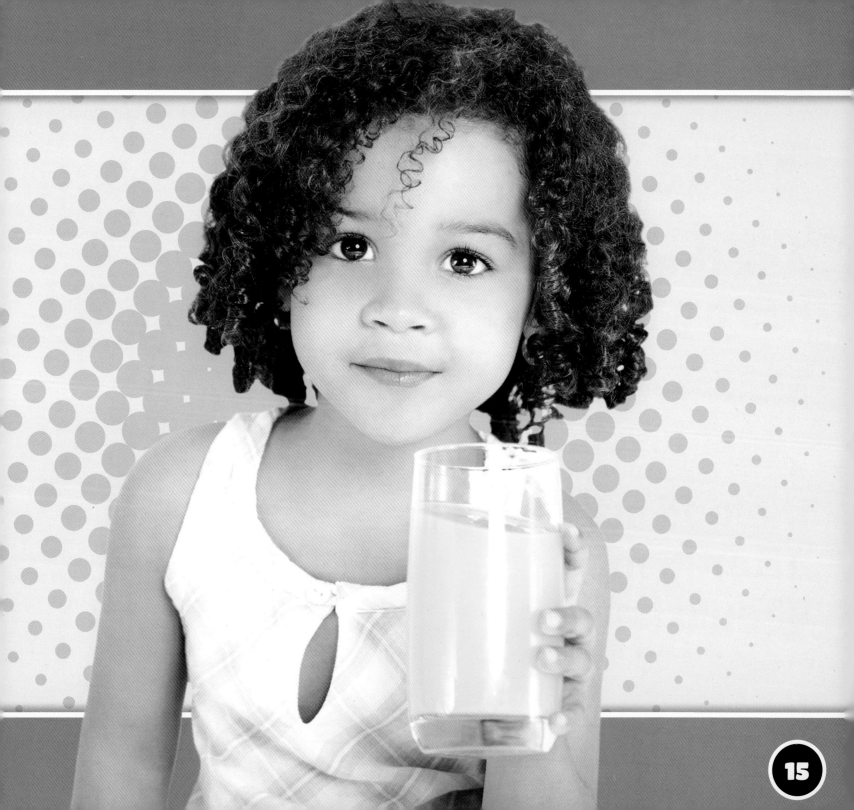

# Test

Ask the person if he or she has a glucose meter.

This machine tests blood sugar levels.

If blood sugar is still low after 15 minutes, the person should have another snack.

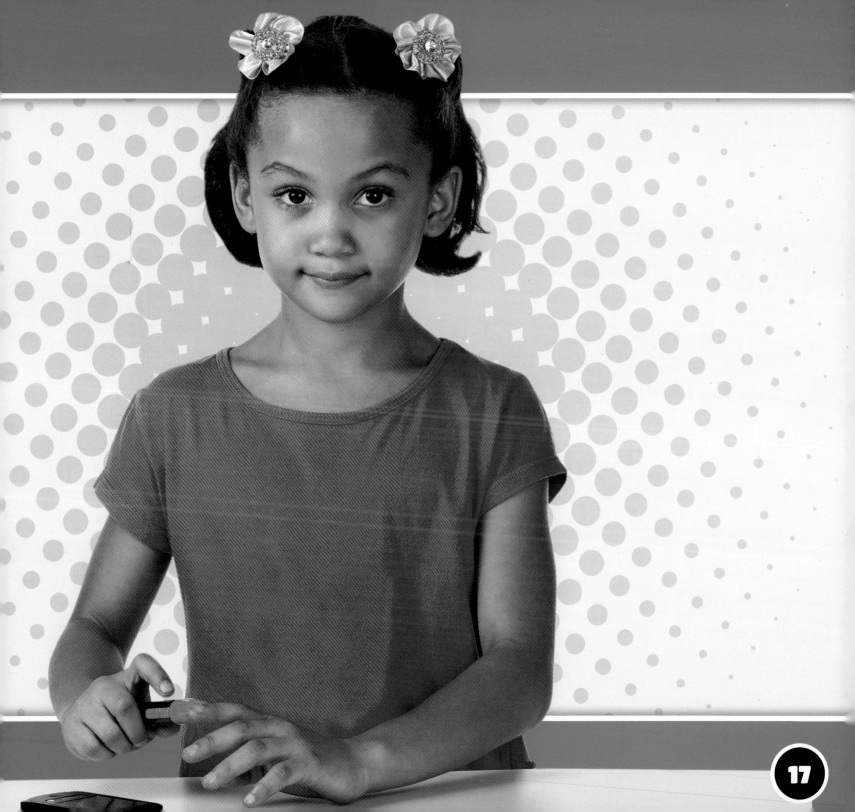

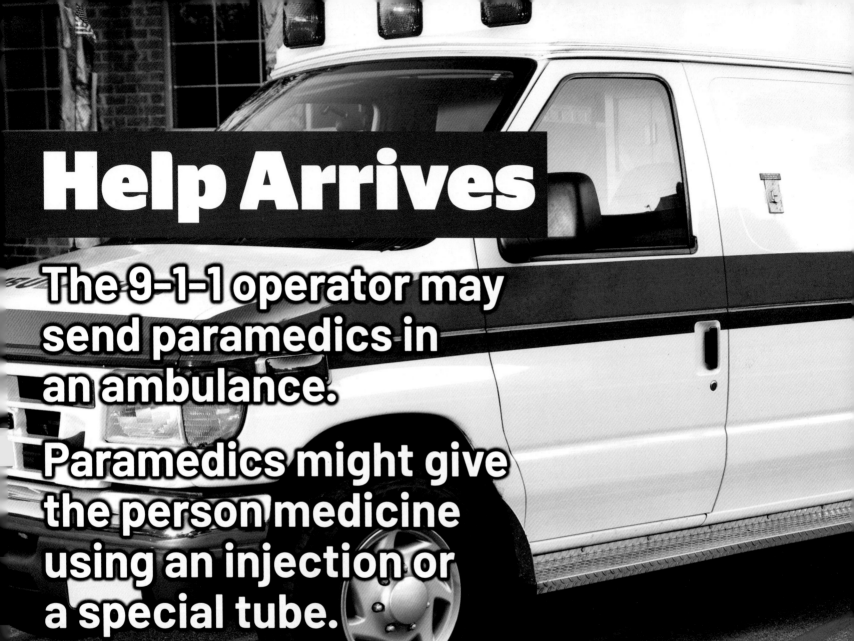

# Help Arrives

The 9-1-1 operator may send paramedics in an ambulance.

Paramedics might give the person medicine using an injection or a special tube.

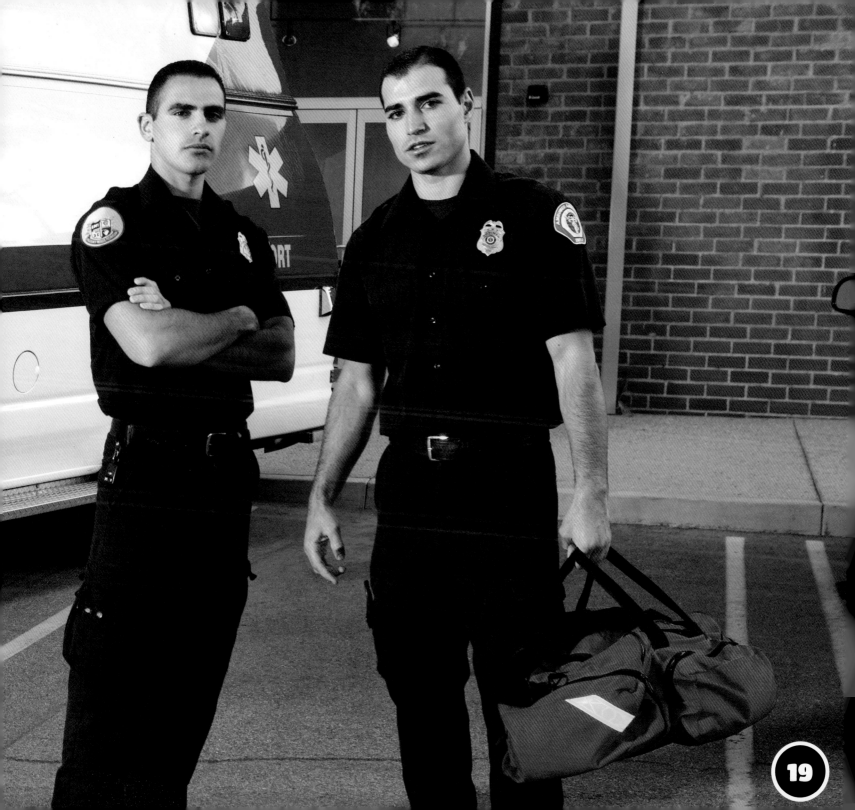

# Preventative Measures

People with diabetes take a medicine called insulin.

It helps their bodies turn sugar from food into energy.

Eating small, regular snacks and meals helps control blood sugar levels.

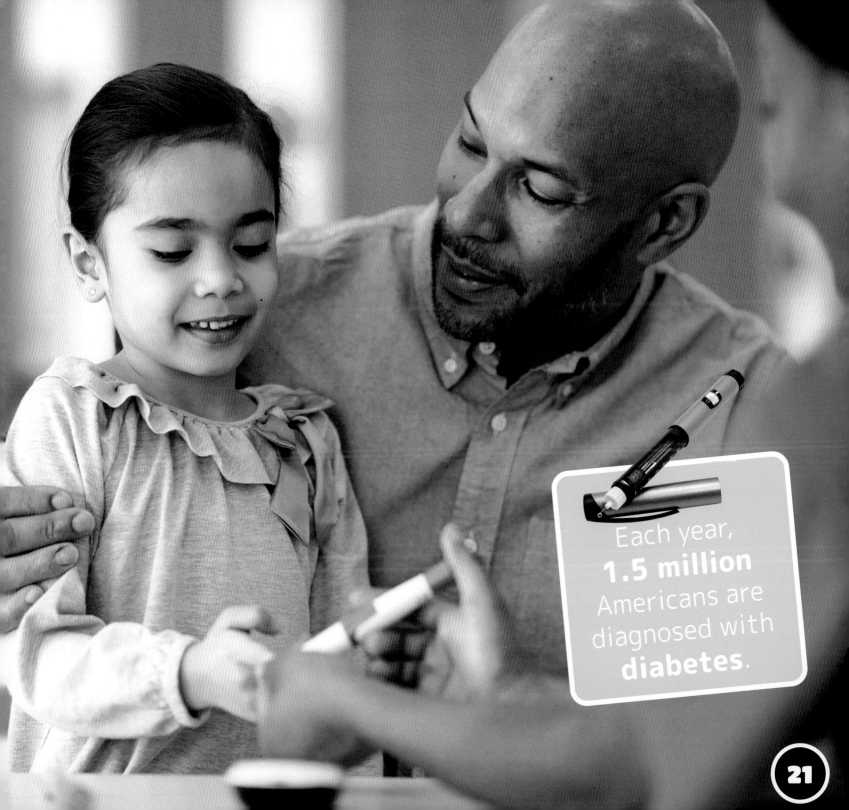

Each year, **1.5 million** Americans are diagnosed with **diabetes**.

# EMERGENCY PROCEDURES

These pages provide detailed information that expands on the emergency found in the book. They are intended to be used by adults as a learning support to help young readers understand the correct responses to each emergency featured in the *In Case of Emergency* series.

**Pages 4–5**

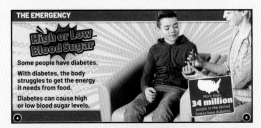

**Some people have diabetes.** Diabetes is a condition where the body does not make or effectively use insulin, a hormone produced by the pancreas. Insulin helps the body process a sugar called glucose. When a person eats food, carbohydrates in the food are broken down into glucose. Insulin allows the cells to absorb the glucose and use it for energy.

**Pages 6–7**

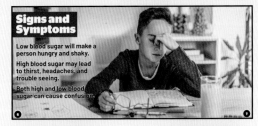

**Low blood sugar will make a person hungry and shaky.** Hypoglycemia, or low blood sugar, is when a person's blood sugar levels drop as a result of not eating enough food or taking too much insulin. Symptoms include hunger, shakiness, fatigue, irritability, sweating, and confusion. Hyperglycemia, or high blood sugar, can be caused by eating the wrong foods or not taking the proper amount of insulin.

**Pages 8–9**

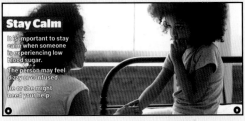

**It is important to stay calm when someone is experiencing a reaction to low blood sugar.** The person experiencing the reaction may be confused and disoriented, so it is especially important for those assisting the patient to stay calm. This will prevent mistakes from being made and can help keep the person having the hypoglycemic attack from becoming agitated.

**Pages 10–11**

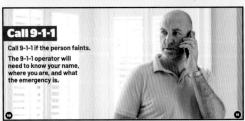

**Call 9-1-1 if the person faints.** A call to 9-1-1 should only be placed in emergency situations. Not all diabetic reactions are severe enough to warrant calling 9-1-1. Call 9-1-1 if a person having the diabetic reaction is unresponsive, unconscious, or having a seizure. In less severe cases, a diabetic reaction can be treated without the assistance of emergency medical services (EMS) or a doctor.

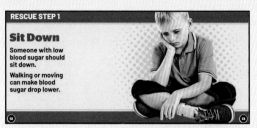

RESCUE STEP 1

**Sit Down**

Someone with low blood sugar should sit down.

Walking or moving can make blood sugar drop lower.

**Someone with low blood sugar should sit down.** Most diabetic reactions are hypoglycemic. The first step to treat hypoglycemia is to have the person sit down. Do not take the person to another location, as walking can make blood sugar levels drop even further. Low blood sugar levels must be treated immediately.

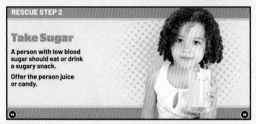

RESCUE STEP 2

**Take Sugar**

A person with low blood sugar should eat or drink a sugary snack.

Offer the person juice or candy.

**A person with low blood sugar should eat or drink a sugary snack.** Give the person suffering from a hypoglycemic attack some sugar to eat or drink. Candy, table sugar, fruit juice, and glucose tablets are possible options. In many cases, diabetics carry sugary snacks or glucose tablets with them. It is important for the person to consume sugar immediately. The person might need to be coaxed into eating or drinking the snack.

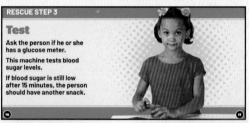

RESCUE STEP 3

**Test**

Ask the person if he or she has a glucose meter.

This machine tests blood sugar levels.

If blood sugar is still low after 15 minutes, the person should have another snack.

**Ask the person if he or she has a glucose meter.** Many diabetics travel with glucose meters on their person. Glucose meters help monitor blood sugar levels. Have the person test his or her blood sugar level every 15 minutes. If the blood sugar is still low after 15 minutes, the person should have another sugary snack.

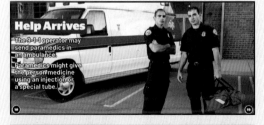

**Help Arrives**

The 9-1-1 operator may send paramedics in an ambulance. Paramedics might give the person medicine using an injection or a special tube.

**The 9-1-1 operator may send paramedics in an ambulance.** When the paramedics arrive, they will assess the situation and monitor the blood sugar levels of the person having the diabetic reaction. Paramedics are trained to administer medication intravenously or through injections to a person having an attack. After administering the medicine, they will reassess the situation. If there is no improvement, they will take the person to a hospital so he or she can be monitored and evaluated by a doctor.

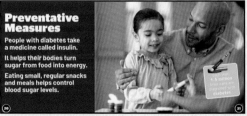

**Preventative Measures**

People with diabetes take a medicine called insulin.

It helps their bodies turn sugar from food into energy.

Eating small, regular snacks and meals helps control blood sugar levels.

**People with diabetes take a medicine called insulin.** Since there is no cure for diabetes, it is up to a person with it to monitor and treat his or her own symptoms. It is important that the person regularly checks his or her blood sugar levels, administering insulin as necessary, and has regular snacks and meals. A snack or sugar may be required before strenuous activity.

# KEY WORDS

**Research has shown that as much as 65 percent of all written material published in English is made up of 300 words.** These 300 words cannot be taught using pictures or learned by sounding them out. They must be recognized by sight. This book contains 59 common sight words to help young readers improve their reading fluency and comprehension. This book also teaches young readers several important content words, such as proper nouns. These words are paired with pictures to aid in learning and improve understanding.

| Page | Sight Words First Appearance | Page | Content Words First Appearance |
|------|------------------------------|------|--------------------------------|
| 4 | can, food, from, get, have, high, it, needs, or, people, some, the, to, with | 4 | blood sugar, body, diabetes, emergency, energy |
| 5 | in, more, states, than | 5 | United States |
| 6 | a, and, both, make, may, will | 6 | confusion, headaches, person, signs, symptoms, thirst |
| 8 | he, help, important, is, might, she, when, your | 10 | address, operator |
| 10 | are, call, if, know, name, what, where, you | 12 | step |
| 12 | down, should | 14 | candy, juice, snack, sugar |
| 14 | eat, take | 16 | glucose meter, machine, minutes |
| 16 | after, another, ask, has, still, this | 18 | ambulance, injection, medicine, paramedics, tube |
| 18 | an, give | 20 | insulin, meals, preventative measures |
| 20 | into, small, their, turn | | |
| 21 | Americans, each, year | | |

Published by AV2
14 Penn Plaza 9th Floor New York, NY 10122
Website: www.av2books.com

Printed in Guangzhou, China
1 2 3 4 5 6 7 8 9 0 24 23 22 21 20

052020
100919

Project Coordinator: Ryan Smith
Art Director: Terry Paulhus

Library of Congress Cataloging-in-Publication Data

Names: Hopkins, Linda K., author.
Title: Diabetes / Linda Hopkins.
Description: New York, NY : AV2, [2021] | Series: In case of emergency | Audience: Ages 5-9 | Audience: Grades 2-3
Identifiers: LCCN 2020014383 (print) | LCCN 2020014384 (ebook) | ISBN 9781791126681 (library binding) | ISBN 9781791126698 (paperback) | ISBN 9781791126704 | ISBN 9781791126711
Subjects: LCSH: Diabetes--Juvenile literature. | Medical emergencies--Juvenile literature.
Classification: LCC RC660.5 .H67 2021 (print) | LCC RC660.5 (ebook) | DDC 616.4/62--dc23
LC record available at https://lccn.loc.gov/2020014383
LC ebook record available at https://lccn.loc.gov/2020014384

Every reasonable effort has been made to trace ownership and to obtain permission to reprint copyright material. The publisher would be pleased to have any errors or omissions brought to their attention so that they may be corrected in subsequent printings.

The publisher acknowledges Getty Images, iStock, and Shutterstock as its primary image suppliers for this title.